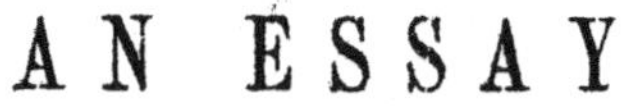

AN ESSAY

ON

HIPPOCRATES,

BY

M. D. KALOPOTHAKES, M. D.

FEBRUARY, 1857.

PHILADELPHIA:
KING & BAIRD, PRINTERS,
1857.

AN ESSAY

ON

HIPPOCRATES,

BY

M. D. KALOPOTHAKES, M. D.

FEBRUARY, 1857.

PHILADELPHIA:
KING & BAIRD, PRINTERS,
1857.

TO THE

VENERABLE REV. R. BAIRD, D.D.

AS A TOKEN OF

RESPECT AND GRATITUDE,

THIS PAMPHLET

IS INSCRIBED BY THE

AUTHOR.

OF MEDICINE BEFORE HIPPOCRATES.

THERE were both physicians and medicine before the time of Hippocrates. The natural tendency or instinct in man to preserve self, and to avoid every thing injurious to health and destructive of life on the one hand, accident, observation, and the analogy of the same circumstances on the other, were the first sources of medicine. So that we may with propriety and truthfulness affirm that it is synchronous with man himself. And, as it would have been with man's appearing upon the face of the earth, and with his immediate descendants, had it not been for the Revelation of God, so it is with the beginning of this science—it is enveloped in the darkness and mystifications of the so called Mythological ages. Osiris, Isis, Thoth, Mercury, Or, Apollo, gods, demigods, and heroes of the Phœnicians, Egyptians and Greeks, constitute the first mythological epoch of medicine, which extends itself down to the time of Esculapius, whose sons Podalirius and Machaon, skilful physicians, accompanied the Greek army against the City of Troy. (Iliad II, 732.)

Two things are worth mentioning concerning the whole of this period. 1. The custom that existed among some ancient nations, and especially the Babylonians, of exposing their sick in the streets, markets and high-ways, for the purpose of ascertaining the curative means from those who might have previously suffered or witnessed similar diseases; and 2. The condition of medicine in Egypt. (See Herod., book II. ch. I. Diod. of Sicily, book II.) By these means materials of empiricism were little by little collected; practical medicine followed these first steps of empiricism according to observation, accident, and analogy; and these at last became the foundations upon which the Greek mind built the science which is designated by the name of medicine.

Among the hero physicians is numbered Chiron the

Centaur, (1350–1370, B. C.) skilled in herbs and the cure of wounds. His disciple was the famous Esculapius, (1321–1343,) who *acquired greater skill in Botany, Practice of medicine and Surgery*, than his teacher Chiron. So great was his reputation, that temples all over Greece were erected and dedicated to him; and, according to the fashion of those times, he himself was declared and adored as the God of medicine. His priests afterwards like those in Egypt practiced medicine to the exclusion of all others, exercising great influence over the masses because of the reputation of this God. The sick who resorted to them for medical counsel and treatment, when restored to health, were in the habit of writing upon tablets the name of the disease from which they had suffered, and the medicament by the use of which they had been cured, and hang them in the temples. On the greater or smaller number of these tablets depended the reputation of the temples which at last became the resort for the cure of all varieties of diseases. These temples that may be justly and properly termed the first hospitals, were denominated *Asclepiia* from Asclepius to whom they were dedicated; and the priests, who were at the same time his vice-gerents in medicine, were called *Asclepiadæ*. They, like the priests of Egypt, monopolized medicine, and transmitted it to posterity by initiating their sons or immediate relations, into the mysteries of the healing art.

In proportion to the spread of this worship of the God of medicine new Asclepiia were erected everywhere in Greece; and in the lapse of time, they were transformed into medical schools, in which, however, none but the relatives of Asclepiadae had tickets of admission.

The most famous of these Asclepiia were those in Rhode, Cyrene in Libya, Cnidos and Cos. The two first, however, died out not long afterwards; but those of Cnidos and Cos were for a long time in great reputation for their illustrious Asclepiadæ, and the rich collections of practical observations, in which the empiric system of medicine of those times consisted. Hippocrates the Great himself, was educated in one of these schools, viz., that of Cos.

Meanwhile the Philosophers commenced to turn their attention to the study of Botany, Anatomy, Physiology, and Hyginics; and, by their long-continued travels through Egypt and elsewhere they acquired an extensive knowledge of empirical medicine. In this way a new set of physicians sprung up, the so called "*Philosopher Physicians*," and medical schools on this new footing were opened. A kind of rivalry thence arose between these and the Asclepiadæ, the consequence of which was the gradual reformation of medicine, the latter being compelled to rend asunder the veil of secrecy that characterized their proceedings, to cast away their impostures and sorceries, to throw open their Asclepiia to the inspection of the world, and to depend upon experience and proof more than upon charms, amulets, incantations and the supernatural aid of Esculapius. The descendants of Nebrus especially; that is, the ancestors of Hippocrates the Great, distinguished themselves in this reformation. Paying their attention to experience and observation, purging their profession from prejudice and deceit, and faithfully following nature both in its normal phenomena and morbid deviations and issues, they greatly assisted in preparing the way for the father of medicine to elevate it from simple, rude, elementary empiricism to a systematic logical science.

From what has been said, it is obvious that medicine developed itself gradually and slowly; that there were both skilful physicians and medical schools before the time of Hippocrates the Great—and that, to use the language of the learned Sprengel (Histoir de la Medicide, Vol. I., p. 215) "we must seek the first traces of logical and epistemonical study of all human learning, neither in Egypt nor in India, neither in Persia, nor in Rome nor Palestine, but beneath the beautiful blue sky of Greece. Its peculiar geographical and topographical position, surrounded by sea, abounding in bays, harbors, and fertile islands, and its sweet, refreshing and invigorating climate, gave strength and developement to the mind, the imagination and the sense of the beautiful; training on the other hand, and the intercourse with the neighboring nations, assisted to a considerable degree to the perfection of different sciences, and especially that of medicine.

OF HIPPOCRATES THE GREAT.

What an uncertainty and doubt there is of the time in which Hippocrates the Great lived, and of the genuineness of the writings that have come down to us under his name, may be demonstrated by the great multitude of conflicting treatises that have been published on this subject, and by the silence of his contemporary writers. Avoiding the hyperbole of both those who accept all, and those who reject all, we shall treat in this essay of Hippocrates of the following topics:—

1st. Whether Hippocrates the Great ever lived, and in what epoch.

2d. Whether he wrote all the books that bear his name, or some of them only, or none at all.

3d. Whether he deserves the appellation of the *Great.*

I. *Did Hippocrates the Great ever live, and in what epoch?*

The first part of this inquiry may be decided by a single glance at the list of the Hippocrateses with which the older writers have furnished us.

There are mentioned in history twenty-three Hippocrateses, of whom seven only were Asclepiadæ physicians of Cos, the following—

1. Hippocrates the son of Gnosidicus the grand-father of Hippocrates the Great.

2. Hippocrates the 2d, the son of Heraclides and Phænareta.

3. Hippocrates the son of Thessalus, against whom, it is supposed by some, Antiphon the orator wrote.

4. Hippocrates the son of Draco.

5 and 6. The two sons of Thymbæus of Cos.

7. Hippocrates the son of Praxianax, a physician of Cos.

Now, the most famous and illustrious of them all, was,

according to historical records, Hippocrates the Second, son of Heraclides and Phænareta; and, on this account he was called Hippocrates *the Great;* and also *the father of medicine;* not because he first invented medicine, but, because he arranged the already existing sporadic and rude materials of medicine into a systematic form.

Respecting the latter part of the inquiry, viz., in what epoch he did live, there is a little difference of opinion.

Plato in his Phædon, speaks of Hippocrates as teaching medicine, ἐπὶ μισθῷ, and as being acknowledged skilful in the observation of nature and in medicine.

Soranus goes even so far as to specify the very year of his birth, by saying that he was born in the first year of the eightieth Olympiad, Μοναρχοῦντος 'Αβριάδα, μηνὸς 'Αγριανοῦ.

Aulus Gallus, (Noct. Att., xxii. 21,) speaking of the Peloponesian war, mentions Hippocrates as being contemporary with Sophocles and Euripides. "Itaque inter haec "tempora nobiles celebresque erant Sophocles ac deinde "Euripides, tragici poetae, and Hippocrates medicus, et "Democritus philosophus, quibus Socrates Atheniensis natu "quidem posterior fuit, sed quibusdam temporibus iisdem "vixerunt."

But the most complete of all historical records we possess of Hippocrates is a biography of his written by one called Pseudo-soranus. *Biography.*

"Hippocrates by birth was of Cos, the son of Heraclides "and Phænareta, tracing his ancestry to Herculis and Esculapius, the twentieth descendant from the first, and the "twenty-ninth from the latter. Eratosthenes, Pherecydes, "Apollodorus, and Arius of Tarsus make mention of his "genealogy. He became a pupil of Heraclides, his own "father, then of Herodicus, and according to some he studied "under Gorgias of Leontini, the orator, and Draco the Abderite, the philosopher. He flourished during the period of "the Peloponesian war, having been born, as says Histomachus in his first book *of the Hippocratean school,* in the "first year of the eightieth Olympiad, during the *monarchia* "of Abriadas, the twentieth of the month of Agrianus according to Sovanus who had searched the archives of Cos, on which account, he says, the inhabitants of Cos offer sacrifices to Hippocrates on this same day until the present time. Having made himself familiar with medicine and the arts and sciences in general, after the death of his parents, he removed from his country, as Andreas slanderously relates in his book on *Medical Genealogy* on account of having set fire to the Hall of Records at Knidos, as others say for the purpose of beholding the customs and manners of various places, and thus qualifying himself in a more diversified manner. But as Soranus of Cos relates, because he had a dream directing him to inhabit Thessaly. In practicing his profession through the whole of Greece, he attained such reputation that he was publicly invited by Perdicas, the King of the Macedonians, who was supposed to be consumptive. After he went to him with Europhond who was older than himself, he noticed that the malady was a mental one; for the King, after the death of his father, Alexander, fell in love with Phila, his mistress, to whom having revealed the matter, since he had observed that whilst she was in sight he was in excitement, he cured the disease and restored the King to health. He was also requested by the Abderites to come to them and cure Democritus, who was thought to be insane, and save the whole city from the pestilence. Besides, when the pestilence made its appearance in the land of the Ilyrian and Pæonian barbarians, and the kings of those countries requested him to come to them, having ascertained from the ambassadors what were the prevailing winds there, he sent them away without accepting the call; and conjecturing that the disease would come to Attica, he foretold it, and thus rendered himself serviceable both to the cities and to his pupils. And so patriotic he was, that when his fame had reached as far as the Persians, and on this account Artaxerxes had through Istanis, the Governor of Hellespont, requested him to come to him, promising him great gifts, he declined "because of his modesty and freedom from avarice, as is "manifest from his letter to Artaxerxes. He saved also his "native city which was about to be attacked by the Athe- "nians by invoking the assistance of the Thessalians, on "which account he obtained signal honors among the inha- "bitants of Cos. So, likewise among the Thessalians, the "Argives, and the Athenians, who publicly initiated him "the second from Herculis, into the Eleusinian mysteries, "enrolled him as a citizen, and granted him and his descen- "dants the privilege of being entertained at the public "expense in the Prytanium. He liberally taught his friends "his profession together with the becoming oath. He died "among the Larissians at the same time that Democritus is "said to have died, according to some, ninety years of age, "according to others eighty-five, according to others one "hundred and four, and according to some one hundred "and nine. He was buried between Gyrton and Larissa; "and his monument is shown to the present day. Upon "this there was for a long time a swarm of honey-bees "making honey, with which the nurses anointing children "that suffered from aphthæ, at the tomb easily cured them."

"In most of his portraits he is represented with his head "covered, as some say, with a hat, as an emblem of nobility "like Ulises and as others say with his cloak; and among "these some suppose that it was done for the sake of come- "liness, since he was bald; others to express that the lead- "ing part of the body should be guarded; others that it was "an evidence of his roving disposition, or of the obscurity of "his writings, or of the necessity of warding off even in health "what is injurious, and others that he placed upon his head the "loose part of his cloak, folding it together in order to enjoy "freedom of his hands."

"Concerning his writings there has been a diversity of "opinion, some having one opinion and others another. "Hence, it is not easy to determine respecting them, on "account of many causes obscuring the decision first, the "title; second, the ability of preserving the same phraseology "third, the fact that the same person writes now vigorously "and at another time more feebly, on account of his age, "and other causes besides these might be given. He was "free from avarice, modest in his deportment, and a lover "of the Greeks, in as much as he cured his countrymen with "all dilligence, so as to deliver whole cities from pestilence, "as has been mentioned, whence, also, he obtained signal "honors, not only among the inhabitants of Cos, but also "among the Athenians and Argives. At his death he left "two sons, Thessalus and Draco, and very many disciples; and "it is said that he left his sons in a most illustrious position."

From these and other testimonies which we forbear mentioning, it is evident that Hippocrates the great was a native of Cos, a descendant of Asclepiadæ, and the son of Heraclides and Phænareta, that his father too, was called Hippocrates, the son of Gnosidicus; that he learned medicine from his father (as it was customary with all the Asclepiadæ to initiate their sons into the mysteries of the healing art) Rhetoric from Georgias of Leodini, and Philosophy from Democritus the Abderite; that he was known at the time of the Peloponesian war, and according to Celsus he was "*vir et arte et fancundia insignis*," that he left his country for the purpose of improving his medical knowledge, that, as is shown from his writings, he travelled through Seythia, Macedonia, Thessaly, the islands of Archipelago, Thasos, Smyrna and Athens; and that he visited the most illustrious Asclepiæ of his time, where he studied both diseases and their therapeutics, and collected the materials upon which he built his system of medicine.

II. Are all the books that have come down to us under the name of Hippocrates his own works, or some of them, or none at all?

Books ascribed to Hippocrates.

1. The Oath.
2. The Law.
3. Of the Art of Medicine.
4. Of the Art of Medicine in former times.

5. Of the Physician.
6. Of Decency and Decorum.
7. Precepts.
8. The Book of Prognostics.
9. On the Humours.
10. On Crises.
11. On Critical Days.
12. Predictions' Book, 1.
13. Predictions' Book, 2.
14. The Coan Prognostics.
15. Of the Nature of Man.
16. Of Generation.
17. Of the Fœtal Nature.
18. Of the Origin of Man.
19. Of the Seventh Month Birth.
20. Of the Eighth Month Birth.
21. Of Superfœtation.
22. Of Dentition.
23. Of the Heart.
24. Of the Glands.
25. Of the Nature of the Bones.
26. Of Airs, Waters, and Localities.
27. Of Flatus.
28. Of Epilepsy.
29. Of Healthy Diet.
30. Of Regimen, books 1, 2, 3.
31. Of Dreams.
32. Of Aliment.
33. Of Diet and Acute Diseases.
34. Of the Different Parts of Man.
35. Of the Use of Liquids.
36. Of Diseases.
37. Of Affections.
38. Of Internal Affections.
39. Of the Diseases of Virgins.
40. Of the Nature of Women.
41. Female Diseases, books 1, 2.

42. Of Barrenness.
43 Of Vision.
44. Of the Office of the Physician.
45. Of Fractures.
46. Of Joints.
47. Of the Reduction of Fractures and Luxations.
48. Of Ulcers.
49. Of Fistulæ.
50. Of Hæmorrhoids.
51. Of Wounds of the Head.
52. Of the Extraction of the Dead Fœtus.
53. Of Dissections.
54. Epidemics, books 1, 2, 3, 4, 5, 6, 7.
55. Of Pestilential Constitution.
56. The Book of Aphorisms.
57. Of Mania.
58. Of Medicines.
59. Of Horse Diseases.
60. Of the Use of Veratrum.
61. Twenty-two Epistles.

Time that spares nothing, revolutions, wars and emigrations, the selfishness and egotism of ancient philosophers and sophists, the conflagration of libraries, and the expensiveness of copying, how much all these causes have contributed to the loss, mutilation, plagarism and spuriousness of the ancient writings before the invention of printing, is already and well known to those who occupy themselves with the history of letters. No wonder, then, if the writings of Hippocrates, too, met with a similar fate. And it seems probable that this took place, especially at the time of the Kings of Pergamus and Egypt. "Πϱὸς ἀλλήλους ἀντιφιλοτιμουμένων πεϱὶ κτήσεως τῶν βιβλίων, (as Galen remarks,) ἡ περὶ τὰς ἐπιγραφὰς καὶ διασκευάς ἦρξατο γίνεσθαι ῥᾳδιουργία." An examination of the writings themselves, however, and a comparison with each other, will at once convince one that they have not all come out of the same hand. All the ancient commentators of Hippocrates without exception and among them Galen who devoted himself particularly to the scrutiny of the Hippocratean writings, declares that most of them were written by writers either anterior or posterior to Hippocrates. He observes that he could distinguish the spurious from the genuine ones from their phraseology, and the theories they advocated; and promises in his commentary on "*Humours*," to write a special work on this point. If he did in fact fulfil his promise, that work like many others is lost. The same author declares that he had seen in the Royal Library of Pergamus manuscripts of Hippocrates' writings that were written three hundred years previous to that time; and this is not improbable; for we can trace historical records of Hippocrates' writings as far back as the time of Aristotle. This point, then, being decided, the question next arises, which of these writings are the genuine writings of Hippocrates the Great?

From the Alexandrian epoch down to the present day there has been a difference of opinion among the Philologists and Critics in regard to the genuine works of Hippocrates. All of them however, both ancient and modern, admit that the following works were written by Hippocrates himself.

1. The first seven books of Aphorisms.
2. The Book of Prognostics.
3. Of Diet and Acute Diseases.
4. The first and third Books of Epidemics.
5. Of Fractures of the Head.

The rest are attributed, some to his sons Thessalus and Draco, some to his son-in-law Polybus, others to Hippocrates the first, and others to others.

III. Does Hipprocrates deserve the appellation of the Great?

If we take into consideration the moral and religious condition of the World and the comparatively dimmed and obscure lights of sciences at the time of Hippocrates; and then peruse the system he was able to form in spite of them all, we would not deny him this title given him by his posterity; for the fewer and more imperfect the means he possessed, the greater must be the cause for our admiration and esteem that he wrote so well. Had he lived in our time with all the means we possess at his disposal for his co-operation, he might have outshone all and every one of the brightest stars that adorn and illuminate the medical horizon. His observing character, his disposition to order and arrangement, and his unprejudiced and sound judgment led him to place the facts he has obtained by his own observation and the experience of his predecessors, on a basis that has heroically borne the large superstructure laid upon it by the investigations of more than two thousand years. Nay, he has done more than that, he has given us such general rules, theories and precepts, that thoug h they admit expansion, shall still hold true as long as earth exists. Who can actually peruse his writings without finding in them a complete encyclopedia of all the elementary knowledge *both practical and theoretical of medicine*, sufficient to evince him of the greatness of *the man?* Who can read his oath without feeling the full power of the noble qualities of his soul, or his prognostics without admiration at the philosophical conclusions to which his close observations had led him? Which of the medical men would not acknowledge the correctness of the axiom-like aphorisms of this great man, and wonder at the almost perfect way of treating dislocations fractures and wounds? What can be added to the advice he gives to the physician, that he should take into consideration the age, sex, temperament, climate, localities, seasons of the year, prevailing epidemics and to sympathies existing between different organs of the system—that he should derive his symptoms from every source; from the countenance, the eyes, the mode of decubitus, the motions of the arms and hands, the talkativeness and silence of the individual, his respiration, the condition of the skin and tongue, watchfulness or somnolency, his excretions of all kinds, such as faces, urine, sweat, crepitus, saliva, sputa, tears &c., both in relation to quantity and quality; and above all that he should endeavor by all means to trace and find out the cause of the disease and cure it? Who can deny this great truth he laid down more than two thousand years ago, viz: that it is not medicine that cures disease, but Nature; and that the physician should employ such means that should strengthen and facilitate its operations to the accomplishment of this end? And yet there are not a few in the medical circle who know but the name of this *man*! And there are many more who unfortunately believe that all they find in the medical books of our day are the achievements of modern times, and that the writings of such men as Hippocrates and Galen are to be considered but as monuments worthy of being preserved in the files of Public Libraries rather than to be taken up and consulted by men so much advanced in the knowledge of medicine!

In closing this brief and imperfect treatise on Hippocrates, I cannot but wish and hope that the day is not far off when some one of the young American physicians would undertake to translate the writings not only of Hippocrates, but also of Galen. The work at first sight appears of little or no importance; but when done it will amply repay him for all his labors, and give to the American medical world the benefit of the experience of those men whom they are taught to respect and admire for their high medical attainments and for the scientific shape they have given to the all-important art—*Medicine.* Before that time, however, we would advise all who occupy themselves with the art of medicine to read the excellent volume of Dr. Coxe on Hippocrates and Galen. We were very much pleased with the accurate outline given by its learned author of Hippocrates and Galen and their writings, and think that it should have a place in the library of every medical man.

www.ingramcontent.com/pod-product-compliance
Lightning Source LLC
LaVergne TN
LVHW020636110826
845149LV00004B/1232

* 9 7 8 1 4 1 8 1 9 0 8 7 3 *